Strength Training Nutrition

7 Key Things To Create The Right Strength Training Diet Plan For You

Jason Scotts

Table of Contents

Copyright

Introduction

Whether you're trying to enhance your performance as an athlete or just attempting to lose weight, including some form of strength training into your exercise regime is crucial. However it's also important you make sure you're following the right sort of strength training diet and nutrition plan to really reap the benefits.

If you aren't eating the right kinds of foods then you won't actually make the most of each strength training session you undertake. However if you aren't sure about what you should being eating and drinking then creating the right sort of plan can be difficult.

There are a few things you need to consider when putting together your eating plan.

1. Providing Your Body with the Right Fuel Is Key

Before you begin any strength training workout you must make sure, not only is your body well nourished, but also well hydrated. This will help to ensure there's enough energy available to provide your bloodstream and muscles with a more effective workout. If you can, eat a pre-workout snack or meal before you begin your exercises.

It's important you choose foods to provide your body with fuel that have plenty of carbohydrates in them as well as provide you with a source of protein. These will help to provide your body with sustained energy.

Some of the things you could consider having before you begin your workout that includes plenty of carbohydrates and protein are as follows:

1. Smoothies. You can make these at home that could include milk, soymilk, and yogurt, fruit or fruit juice in them.

2. Low fat cheese with crackers.

3. Any carbohydrate based energy or granola bars. You may want to consider trying to make your own.

4. Plain yogurt with fruit and ½ a whole grain bagel, roll or slice of bread with nut butter.

Not only do you need to eat right you need to make sure you're keeping your body well hydrated. One way to do this is by drinking a glass of water with every meal or snack you have before you begin your workout. Ideally you should drink two to three glasses of water at least 2 to 3 hours before your workout is due to commence.

2. Make Sure You Provide Your Muscles With Fuel To Help Them Recover

As well as providing your body with the nutrients it needs before you start working out, you also need to provide it with what it needs after you've finished your workout. Studies clearly show that eating the right sorts of carbohydrates and protein within 30 minutes of finishing your workout is the most effective way to help restore the levels of amino acids and carbohydrates in your muscles.

Not only should you eat 30 minutes after your workout to help rebuild muscle energy, but again a further 2 hours after completing your workout.

It isn't only about eating the right sorts of foods; you must also make sure you're drinking plenty of fluids. After finishing your workout make sure you drink at least 2 glasses of water to replenish your system.

3. Building Muscle – Protein versus Carbohydrates

When it comes to nutrition, most athletes tend to eat meals that include high levels of protein. It was believed that a high amount of protein builds muscle bulk. This has since been found not to be true. However, increasing your daily protein levels does help to rebuild muscle.

Carbohydrates actually play a very important role as part of your strength-training program. Unlike protein, which helps to build muscles, your muscles need carbs to provide energy when exercising them.

Although eating sufficient amounts of protein helps to build and protect your muscles, if you eat too much it won't help you in any way to gain muscle or muscle strength.

Through this book you will get to know how feeding and watering your body regularly will help you to achieve the results you desire. You'll also learn how important a well-developed strength training diet and nutritional plan is to helping you to build up strength.

Chapter 1 – Why Your Diet Must Include Protein?

It's important when working out you make sure you eat the right kinds of foods to ensure your body gets the energy it needs. If you spend time focusing on creating the right kind of strength training diet and nutrition plan, you'll be making sure your body is getting all the nutrients, vitamins, minerals and proteins it needs to provide it with fuel to complete such intense workouts.

Before you actually start work on creating the right diet and nutrition plan you need to understand the difference between a strength training diet plan and one for losing weight. Normally when people hear the word diet they jump straight to the conclusion it needs to be low in fat and carbs.

When it comes to a strength training diet, although it's similar to that for losing weight, there is one fundamental difference. In order to build more muscle you need a diet that provides your body with more energy. In fact in order to achieve such goals the diet you need to follow is quite different from what you would follow to lose weight.

Why protein plays such an important role in your strength-training regime.

Proteins

Protein is the building block of muscles. Including plenty of protein in your diet not only helps to make your muscles stronger but also helps to ensure you complete your workout more effectively.

What you need to remember though, is over doing the protein won't make you gain muscle quicker neither will it make them bigger. In fact what happens is the protein your body needs will go into repairing the muscle and the rest will be flushed away.

How to Calculate the Protein You Need

When you are doing any kind of strength training you need to be aiming at eating between 1.2 and 1.5 grams of protein each day for each kilogram you weigh. For example, say you weigh 58kg then you need to be eating between 70 and 87 grams of protein each day. 1 gram protein = 4 calories. So the total number of calories you'll be eating when you consume 70 grams of protein is 280.

Choosing Which Type of Protein to Eat

It depends on what food you enjoy. You'll find both meat and vegetarian dishes provide you with your daily protein requirements. However protein is more abundant in meat such as beef, chicken and pork as well as fish. But be aware that although these do contain the most complete proteins to be found in food they also contain high numbers of calories as well.

You also need to consider there are 8 essential amino acids your body needs in order to function properly as well as to help build muscle. That's why it's important you make sure you include eggs and dairy products such as milk and yogurt in your diet.

So How Do You Get The Protein You Need?

There are several ways in which you can get all the protein your muscles needs into your diet. These are:

1 – Food

There are plenty of foods that contain protein.

The kinds of foods you must make sure you're eating on a daily basis are as follows:

1. Lean Steak (with as little or no fat as possible)
2. Eggs
3. Chicken Breast (without the skin)
4. Fish (any type)

Here's a typical menu:

1. Breakfast

In a pan scramble some egg whites with a few vegetables and then top off with a slice of whole-wheat toast.

Great vegetables to include are tomatoes and mushrooms.

2. Lunch

Have either tuna or lean meat inside a whole-wheat tortilla with some grilled vegetables or a fresh green salad.

3. Dinner

For your evening meal why not grill or bake a piece of chicken breast, lean steak or fish and serve it with lightly steamed vegetables and brown rice. Not only will this meal provide you with plenty of protein, but also plenty of healthy nutrients and carbs your body needs.

4. Snacks

Of course you may feel hungry during the day, when feeling peckish eat fruit, vegetables, low fat cheese or some non-fat yogurt.

2 – Protein Shakes

As the name suggests these are made up of various types of proteins your body's able to absorb. Normally they come in powder form and you add to either milk or juice. These particular shakes provide your body with large amounts of protein that'll help to ensure muscles get repaired more effectively after you've completed one of your very strenuous strength training workouts.

Whatever you do, don't replace meals with protein shakes. Keep the shakes for after your workout and PART of your diet.

However although protein shakes take very little time to prepare you need to be wary about using them as they may contain substances that aren't listed on the container. These may actually prove detrimental to your health and of course detrimental to you achieving your goals. Nonetheless if you make sure you read the ingredients clearly then you shouldn't have a problem.

3 – Meal Replacements

In some ways these are similar to protein shakes but they do contain a lot more nutrients and other ingredients in them such as fibre and act like a full-blown meal.

Although these will provide your body with the essential nutrients, carbohydrates, proteins and vitamins it needs, you still have to eat some food as well. Meal replacements are a good way to give your body what it needs if you don't have the time to eat a proper meal.

The above ways can help to provide your body with what it needs to help build muscle and lose weight. However creating your own diet plan does depend on your own particular tastes and how many calories you need to consume. What's important to remember is you need to not only be consistent with what you eat but how you eat it as well.

Certainly when it comes to creating the right kind of strength training diet and nutrition plan it needs to be centered around your own specific needs and goals. If you have any doubt about your plan, then go speak with your doctor or a nutritionist.

Chapter 2 – Foods You Need To Eat To Provide Protein

When using weights you need to make sure you're eating foods that help your muscles recover more effectively and that's why protein is important in your diet.

So Why Make Sure You Include Plenty Of Foods Rich In Protein?

The main aim of proper protein intake is to ensure you eat adequate amounts throughout the day, remembering to eat more after a workout. Those who eat protein after a strength training session are helping to restore the muscle tissue that's been stressed when working out.

You may not see any differences initially but over time, as you start to build strength, your body will become much leaner. Rather than relying on supplements to provide your body with the protein it needs you should be consuming as many foods that contain protein as possible.

Eating these foods help your muscles to recover better and provide your body with other minerals and vitamins it needs in order to function effectively.

Include:

1. Lean Beef

This provides your body with an ideal source of protein. If you can, you should look at eating around 20 to 30 grams of lean beef following any workout.

2. Eggs & Egg Whites

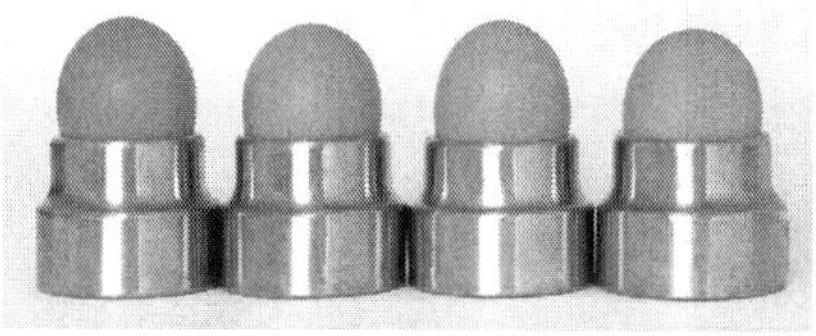

This food is one of the highest quality protein sources available to you. Plus they also contain plenty of amino acids, which is crucial for helping to build up healthy muscle.

3. Tofu

As well as containing high levels of protein this vegetarian food also contains large amounts of fats that are good for your heart and free from cholesterol.

4. Quinoa (Keenwah)

This particularly mild grain has quite a pleasant chewy texture and is very high in protein. In fact the levels of protein found in this particular food are even higher than what's found in normal whole grain products. You can add it to a stew or put in a salad.

5. Legumes

The kinds of legumes you must include in your strength training diet are lentils, beans and peas. All of which are packed full of protein and carbs. Lentils also contain high levels of Vitamin B, which are great for helping to boost metabolism.

Also lentils contain plenty of magnesium and iron, which aren't only good for your bones but also to ensure your body produces plenty of healthy red blood cells.

6. Skinless Chicken Breast

This particular food provides you with one of the leanest sources of protein your body needs. Just 3 ounces of skinless chicken breast is going to provide your body with 94 calories, 20 grams of protein and 1 gram of fat.

7. Fish Rich in Omega 3

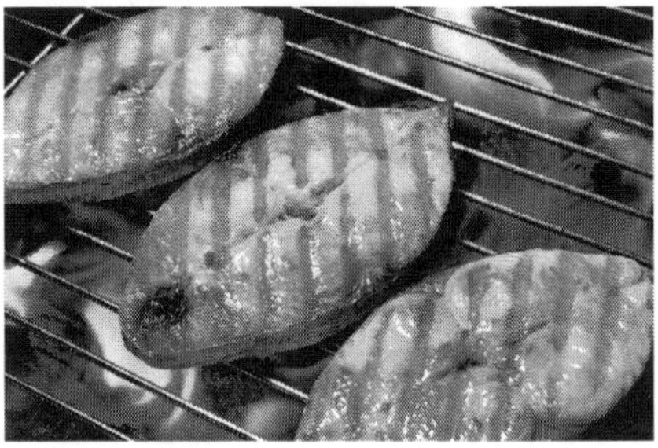

Fish contains good levels of protein and contains very little saturated fat, which leads to arteries becoming clogged. Also eating fatty fish that has high levels of Omega 3 can help to bring levels of triglyceride in the body down.

One particular fish you should include in your diet is Cod, as not only does it contain around 135 grams of protein for each 3-ounce serving but also contains selenium. This is an enzyme that has very strong antioxidant powers, which will help to improve the function of enzymes in the body.

Chapter 3 – Your Diet Shouldn't Only Contain Protein

The diet you need to follow must contain plenty of carbs to provide your body with the energy it needs as well as moderate amounts of fat.

When it comes to creating the perfect diet and nutrition plan for your strength-training regime you need to be aware of one thing. Over time your energy needs are going to change dependent on how much training you do, how often you do it and what your overall goals are.

If your goal is to lose fat, then your diet will be different to that of someone wanting to gain muscle.

So what components make for a healthy balanced diet?

Carbohydrates

If you don't include carbohydrates into your diet then your body will start to use the protein you've eaten to provide it with energy. Plus eating enough carbs daily can also ensure you won't tire so easily when working out, as well as helping to reduce the risk of causing an injury to yourself.

It's important when you start creating your strength training diet and nutrition plan that you aim to eat between 2.3 and 3.6 grams of carbs for each pound you weigh.

The kinds of foods that offer you a good supply of carbs are the following:

1. Whole grains such as whole wheat bread, pasta, brown rice and quinoa
2. Fruit
3. Dairy
4. Sports Bars and Drinks

Fat

Although the fat you're eating won't be used as a primary source of energy when working out, it's still important you include foods containing fat into your diet. It's a very important macronutrient your body needs and will help to provide energy to your body when doing low or moderate intensity exercises. Plus fat also helps to insulate your organs.

When it comes to creating the right kind of diet for your strength-training regime, make sure it includes enough fat to provide around 20 to 35% of the energy your body needs. I would highly recommend you avoid following a diet low in fat as this can lead to your body not being provided with certain nutrients it needs and will affect how well you perform.

The kinds of foods that'll provide you with the fat you need are as follows:

1. Fish
2. Nuts
3. Nut Oil
4. Seeds
5. Vegetable Oils and Vegetable Oil Based Spreads

A Word of Warning

It's important you limit your intake of saturated fat found in full fat dairy products such as butter, high fat cheese and whole milk as well as the fat found in animal products such as lard and cuts of meat that are highly marbled.

But you also need to remember both meat and dairy products provide your body with nutrients and energy so go for the much leaner options available. Go for milk that is either low in fat or fat free, eat low fat cheeses and enjoy meat that has been trimmed. As well as providing your body with much less saturated fat they also provide your body with the nutrients and protein it needs.

Furthermore it's important you make sure you reduce the amount of food that contains "trans fats" such as hydrogenated oil.

Chapter 4 – Things To Consider To Create The Perfect Diet

When it comes to creating the perfect strength training diet and nutrition plan there are numerous things that need to be considered. In this chapter we'll look at some tips you may find useful to help you to create the right diet and nutrition plan that will help to meet your particular strength training needs.

Most people when trying to design the perfect diet and nutrition plan will add up their daily meals then divide them by the amount of fat, protein and carbohydrates they include. Then multiplying these percentages by what their daily calorie requirement is needed. The problem with doing this is it leaves them feeling somewhat confused as it seems to state they are in fact eating too much.

Furthermore matters become even more complicated when it seems most fitness professionals don't actually agree on what's right for you. Although they may agree on some things such as the need to ensure you're drinking plenty of water to keep the body hydrated, it seems this is the only thing they agree on.

When it comes to you eating fat, protein and carbohydrates you'll find each nutritionist will have views that differ. However one thing I've learnt, is although their opinions may differ somewhat, they aren't so different you won't be able to take suggestions from different sources.

Certainly the differences they do recommend are very subtle ones, so what this means is if your current diet plan isn't proving to be as effective as you'd like, then making small changes can help you get on track with achieving your goals.

However when it comes to starting a diet and nutrition plan that's going to complement your strength training program there are certain guidelines you need to follow.

Although these guidelines are useful I would still highly recommend you speak to a nutritionist or your physical trainer to help evaluate your diet so you're able to create one that's going to be more effective for you.

One of the most important things to remember when it comes to creating your plan is to remember you're using strength training to help you lose fat whilst increasing muscle mass and energy. Certainly the guidelines I offer below are actually going to help simplify the process of creating such a plan.

Guideline 1 – Meals per Day

Ideally you should be eating every two to three hours during the day. Therefore on a daily basis you should be eating between 6 and 8 small meals. By eating regularly you're ensuring your body's being supplied with energy constantly. Plus eating small meals regularly reduces the risk of wanting to binge because you're feeling hungry.

It's important to make sure any meals you have before your workout are eaten at least 60 minutes beforehand. Plus you should be aiming to eat another meal at least an hour or two after your workout.

Guideline 2 – How to Determine What Your Meal Should Be Made Up Of

Generally speaking it's acceptable when undertaking any form of strength training to follow a low fat diet. However, how little fat you consume is certainly up for debate. There are some nutritionists and trainers who believe each meal should contain less than 10% fat, whilst others believe that 10% or more is acceptable. In fact in some cases there are trainers and nutritionists who believe including 30% fat in each meal is okay.

However fat shouldn't be the only thing your meal should include, it's also important it includes adequate amounts of protein and carbohydrates as well. When creating a meal, around 20 to 30% should be made up of protein whilst the other 40 to 60% should be made up of carbohydrates.

If you find working in percentages difficult then use this method instead. For each pound you weigh you should be eating 1 to 1.5 grams of protein and 2 to 3 grams of carbohydrates.

Guideline 3 – How to Determine Your Daily Calorie Goal

When wanting to increase muscle mass, you must eat more calories than your body's going to burn. If you're quite active already then to determine how many calories you should be consuming daily, you times your current body weight by 20. This will provide you with a fairly reliable indicator of how many calories you need to be consuming each day. I weigh around 128lbs therefore my daily calorie intake should be around 2,560.

Guideline 4 – Snack Wisely

When it comes to snacking you need to be careful about what you eat. Today there are plenty of snack bars available that are suitable for those doing strength training. However with so many to choose from deciding which is the right one can prove quite a challenge.

The best piece of advice I can give you about choosing the right snack bar is to go for ones where the carbs to protein ratio is between 2:1 and 4:1. Plus never eat any bars that contain over 200 calories.

Guideline 5 – Keep Yourself Hydrated

Keeping hydrated is important for several reasons. Not only does it help to replace fluid lost as you workout, but will help to keep the cartilage in your joints hydrated as well. Plus drinking plenty of water will reduce the chances of you causing harm to these areas of your body.

Although water is a great way to ensure your body remains hydrated consuming certain sports drinks can prove beneficial as well, especially during and after you've worked out. These drinks contain glucose, which can provide you with the additional energy your body needs.

On average you should be looking to drink no less than 8 glasses of water each day on top of what you should drink whilst working out. Each glass of water you drink should contain no less than 227ml (8 fluid ounces) in each one.

Guideline 6 – Don't Restrict Yourself

Sometimes sticking with a diet can prove difficult because they can be quite restrictive with regards to what you eat. However if you want to avoid such a situation then don't be afraid to take one day a week off and eat what you want.

Guideline 7 – Focus On Food Quality

In order for muscle mass to be increased, will of course require you to increase how many calories you consume on a daily basis. Although consuming sugary soft drinks along with foods dense in fat and calories can help you to gain weight they won't actually help increase muscle mass. This is because these foods contain properties that cause them to be absorbed by the body and stored as fat.

Instead you must make sure you include foods in your diet that contain high quality nutrients instead. The kinds of foods that are more acceptable to help increase your calorie intake but will help increase muscle mass are whole grains and starchy vegetables along with nuts, seeds, avocados and oils such as extra virgin olive oil and canola oil.

Always eat fresh foods rather than processed. Fresh foods contain vital vitamins, minerals and nutrients your body needs. Not only will you find you're able to meet and maintain your physical goals when working out, but also protect your body because your immune system is strengthened.

Guideline 8 – Avoid Fad Diets

There are numerous fad diet programs and products available that all claim to help promote muscle mass whilst providing you with a much leaner physique. However any reputable nutritionist and fitness professional will tell you programs and products like these should be avoided at all costs.

As well as being expensive, these programs and products tend to be completely ineffective and can lead to you suffering from some very dangerous side effects that could pose a serious risk to your health. As you've already seen from above the most effective way to increase muscle mass and gain a much leaner physique is through following a diet that's rich in nutrients and provides your body with the calories it needs.

Guideline 9 – Set Yourself Realistic Goals

Although making changes to your diet and lifestyle can help improve muscle mass whilst reducing body fat some people find it harder than others. This is because other factors play a role in how effective such diets can be.

When it comes to setting yourself goals, rather than aiming to be a certain size or body shape you should be aiming to improve how toned your muscles become. By doing this you're more likely to find reaching your goals a lot easier.

Guideline 10 – Include Supplements Whenever Possible

There are only a number of supplements you'll need to take to actually see the results you desire. The supplements you should consider taking are as follows:

1. Fish Oil

This particular supplement will help to support your metabolism as well as provide a number of other health benefits. On a daily basis you should be looking to take at least 3 grams of fish oil. Make sure it's a fish oil supplement that contains at least 30% Omega 3.

2. Multi Vitamins

You should either invest in a good multi vitamin supplement or a green powder supplement. This will help to ensure your body's getting enough minerals and vitamins it needs in order to work effectively.

3. Creatine

Taking Creatine everyday helps to prevent muscle loss whilst helping to boost your performance and help your muscles recover more effectively. However be aware it can cause water to be retained by your muscles.

4. Whey Protein

Whey protein is a must especially after you've finished a workout to help your muscles recover from the stress and strain they've been placed under. It's also beneficial in other ways especially when consumed occasionally during the day as it can help to increase the production of protein in the body.

Chapter 5 – Sample Diet & Nutrition Plan

Below is a sample diet plan to help you create your own but before I do that you need to consider these three things:

1. You should aim for around 30 to 50% of your calories coming from eating carbs, with the majority of these being eaten around 0 to 6 hours after you've finished your workout. As for the rest of your calorie intake, make sure around 30 to 40% comes from eating lean sources of protein and the final 20 to 30% comes from consuming good fats.
2. You should make sure you divide your intake of protein up roughly between every meal you eat.
3. Around 2/3 to ¾ of carbs you consume should be eaten prior to your workout and the rest up to 4 to 6 hours after a workout.

My Sample Diet & Nutrition Plan

Breakfast

Breakfast should account for around 15% of the total number of calories you consume in any given day. Your breakfast should be made up of the following:

1/3 Starchy Carbohydrates – Oatmeal, Whole Wheat Bread etc.
2/3 Protein – Eggs, Milk or Lean Meat
1 Spoonful Of Good Fats – Fish Oil, Olive Oil, Nuts etc.
Some Fruit or Vegetables
Water or Green Tea

Lunch & Dinner

These meals should contain the following:

1/3 Starchy Vegetables and/or Fruits - Greens, Sweet Potato, Salad etc.
2/3 Lean Protein – Lean Meat

Spoonful of Good Fats – Fish Oil, Olive Oil, Nuts etc.
Any Other Fruit and Vegetables
Water Or Green Tea

All Other Pre & Post Workout Meals

Remember when eating after a workout these meals should be consumed 4 to 6 hours after it's been completed.

1/3 Starchy Vegetables and/or Fruit – Greens, Sweet Potato, Salad etc.
2/3 Lean Protein – Lean Meat
Spoonful of Good Fats – Olive Oil, Fish Oil, Nuts etc.
Fresh Vegetables and Fruit
Water or Green Tea

Pre Workout Nutrition

Although there isn't any need to include this within your diet plan it will help you to reap the benefits and achieve your goals more effectively.

You should try to include the following.

1. 30 to 40 grams of Fast Absorbing Carbohydrates - Sucrose, Dextrose or Maltodexin.
2. 5 to 15 grams of whey or BCAA powder

Post Workout Nutrition

These should be consumed as soon after your workout as possible:

1. 20 to 40 grams of Whey Protein
2. 40 to 80 grams of Fast Absorbing Carbohydrates - Sucrose, Dextrose or Maltodexin
3. 1 to 2 grams of BCAA
4. 1 to 2 grams of Glutamine

Meal - 1 to 2 Hours after Workout

This will help to ensure energy levels are kept at optimum amounts as well as helping to boost your metabolism. The meal you eat 1 to 2 hours after a workout should include the following:

1. ½ Starchy Carbohydrates – Whole Grains, Pasta, Whole Grain Bread, Oats, Baked Potato etc.
2. ½ Lean Protein – Egg Whites, Tuna or Any Other Fish, Lean Red Meat, Skimmed Milk etc.
3. Minimal Amounts Of Good Fats
4. Fruit & Vegetables
5. Water or Green Tea

Meal - 3 to 4 Hours after Workout

Again as with the previous meal plan this one will help to keep energy at optimum levels. The meal you eat should be comprised of the following:

1. ½ Starchy Carbohydrates – Whole Grains, Pasta, Whole Grain Bread, Oats, Baked Potato etc.
2. ½ Lean Protein – Egg Whites, Tuna or Any Other Fish, Lean Red Meat, Skimmed Milk etc.
3. Minimal Amounts Of Good Fats
4. Fruit & Vegetables
5. Water or Green Tea

Meal - 4 to 6 Hours after Workout

Again you want to be eating foods that'll keep your energy levels up and also help your muscles to recover. This meal should be made up of the following components.

1. 1/3 Starchy Carbohydrates – Whole Grains, Pasta, Whole Grain Bread, Oats, Baked Potato etc.
2. 2/3 Lean Protein – Lean Red Meat, Egg Whites, Tuna or Other Fish, Skimmed Milk etc.
3. Spoonful of Good Fats

Meal to Eat Before Going to Bed

If you don't eat this meal then the chances of your muscles recovering properly is greatly reduced. The meal you should be eating just before you go to bed each night should include the following:

1. 1 Cup Skimmed Milk
2. ½ Scoop Whey Protein
3. ½ Scoop of Casein Protein
4. 2 Cups Skimmed Milk & ½ Scoop Whey Protein

All the information provided above is actually based upon solid scientific principles and are being practiced by many experts today. The principles I've shown you above are ones that will work for anyone and the sample plan I've provided is one which will help you to achieve a much better looking body.

Chapter 6 – Strength Training Diet & Nutrition Recipes

Breakfast Recipes

Recipe 1 – Spicy Scrambled Eggs

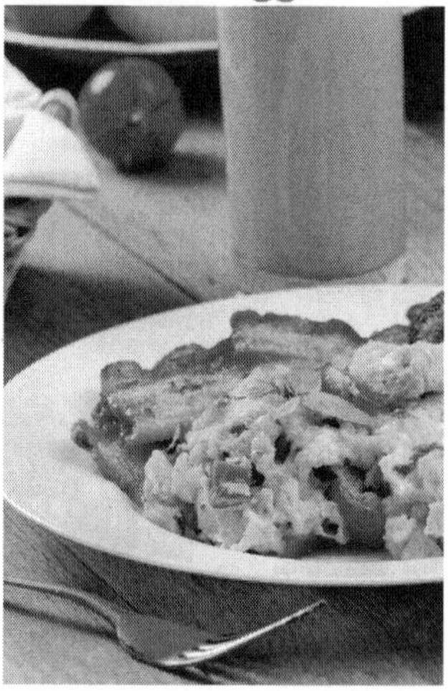

Fed up with eating boring scrambled eggs, then you'll find this recipe really does help to spice them up. Plus this recipe will ensure you're getting a good amount of protein into your diet.

This particular recipe contains 507 calories, 50 grams of protein, and 34 grams of carbs and 19 grams of fat.

Ingredients

2 Large Whole Eggs
4 Egg Whites
¼ Onion – Finely Chopped
1 Whole Red Chilli – Finely Chopped
1 Garlic Clove – Finely Chopped
50 grams Cottage Cheese
Pinch Mixed Herbs
Serve this dish with 2 slices of whole brown bread.

Instructions

Step 1 - Spray a small non stick frying pan with a small amount of olive oil cooking spray. Ensure the entire pan is evenly coated.

Step 2 - In a small mixing bowl place together the 2 whole eggs and the 4 egg whites. Now whisk until the egg yolks and whites are thoroughly combined.

Step 3 – To the eggs add the ¼ onion, the clove of garlic and the chilli. Mix these ingredients thoroughly together.

Step 4 – Add the cottage cheese and herbs and again whisk until all are fully combined together.

Step 5 – Place the oiled frying pan on to the hob on a moderate heat and pour in the contents of the mixing bowl. Make sure you gently stir the contents poured into the frying pan to scramble the eggs.

Step 6 – Just before you're due to remove the eggs from the heat, toast the two slices of whole brown bread and once it's ready, place it and the scrambled eggs on to a plate and enjoy.

NB: Instead of scrambling the eggs you could make them into an omelette. Then serve the omelette on some spinach. Not only does it add a little more color to the dish but also a little more flavor and some additional vitamins your body needs.

Recipe 2 – Pumpkin Spice Pancakes

This particular recipe contains moderate amounts of protein but high levels of carbs.

In total you will get 460 calories from this meal. The pancakes are made up of 25 grams of protein, 75 grams of carbs and 7 grams of fat.

Ingredients

80 grams of Old Fashioned Oats
4 Egg Whites

150 grams of Libby's Solid Packed Canned Pumpkin (If you cannot get hold of Libby's any solid packed canned pumpkin will do)
1 Tablespoon Cinnamon
¼ Cup of Splenda or Stevia or No Calorie Sweetener
1 Teaspoon Baking Powder

Instructions

Step 1 – Pre heat the skillet or griddle on a medium heat.

Step 2 – Whilst the griddle or skillet is heating up grind the oats into a powder using either a coffee grinder or a blender.

Step 3 – Place the ground oats into a large mixing bowl and add the other dry ingredients (cinnamon, non calorie sweetener and baking powder).

Step 4 – Next separate the egg whites from the yolks and mix these together with the canned pumpkin. The canned pumpkin you need be using should have an apple sauce like consistency as this makes it easier to mix with the eggs.

Step 5 – Now take the egg and pumpkin mix and pour this into the bowl with the dry ingredients and mix thoroughly together. If you are finding the mixture a little too thick for your liking then add some water. By adding around a ¼ cup of water to the mixture will help to not only loosen the mixture up but to make an additional 1 or 2 pancakes for you.

Step 6 – Spray the skillet or griddle with some non-stick spray then scoop around a ¼ of a cup of the mixture onto the skillet or griddle.

Step 7 – When you see light bubbles starting to form and the edges of the pancakes start to become firm it will be ready to flip.

Step 8 – Once the pancakes are cooked on both sides, serve and enjoy. You can top these with whatever you like. As these taste quite sweet anyway you won't need to add any additional topping such as honey or maple syrup to them. They are in fact perfect by themselves.

NB: If you'd like to add more carbs to this recipe you can do so by adding some milk rather than water to the mixture. Also if you want to add a little more protein then scoop some vanilla protein powder into the mixture.

Recipe 3 – Banana & Oats Protein Shake

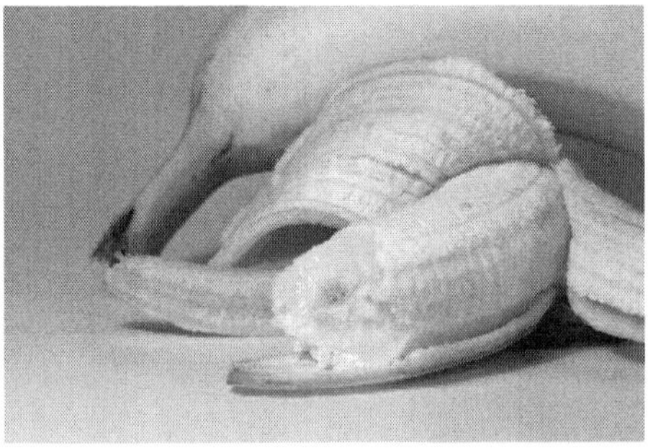

This is a very quick and nutritious shake you can enjoy for breakfast when you don't have much time. You can add any flavor protein powder to this recipe you like.

The amount of ingredients in this recipe makes one complete protein shake. Each shake you drink contains 554 calories, of which 59 grams is protein, 68.2 grams is carbs and 6.1 grams is fat.

Ingredients

8 Fluid Ounces Skimmed Milk
1 Banana
½ Cup Oats
2 Scoops Of Any Flavor Whey Protein Powder You Like

Instructions

Step 1 – Take two scoops of flavored whey protein powder and combine this with all the other ingredients in a blender.

Step 2 – Now turn the blender on and keep it on until the ingredients have become smooth in texture.

Step 3 - Once thoroughly blended together pour into a glass and enjoy.

Lunch Recipes

Recipe 1 – Healthy Chilli

You can make this particular recipe using either lean ground beef or turkey. The recipe below provides you with a total of 10 servings. Each serving contains 488 calories and each serving is made up of 36.8 grams of protein, 51 grams of carbs and 15.4 grams of fat.

By making such a large amount you have several meals available to you over the coming weeks as it freezes really well. Separate into individual portions before you freeze.

Ingredients

2lbs of Lean Ground (80%) Beef or Turkey
1 Tin Stewed Tomatoes
1 Tin Tomato Puree
1 Tin of Corn
1 Tin of Kidney Beans
1 Tin of Garbanzo Beans
1 Tin of Black Beans
1 Tin of Pinto Beans
1 Tin of White Beans
Salt & Pepper To Taste

Instructions

Step 1 – Brown the beef or turkey over a moderate heat.

Step 2 – Now take the browned meat and place in a soup kettle or large saucepan with all the other ingredients mentioned above. Although this recipe calls for 5 cans of certain beans don't be afraid to mix and match if there are certain beans you don't like or aren't able to get hold of.

Step 3 – Season the mixture with salt and pepper and allow cooking until all the ingredients are heated through completely.

Step 4 – Add water if needed, especially if you notice the chilli is a little too thick for your liking.

NB: If you want you can add diced jalapenos or green chilli's to give it even more of a kick. Furthermore you can add any ranch dress seasoning you like or a jar of your favorite salsa.

Recipe 2 – Salsa Chicken Quinoa

As well as being a very simple and tasty meal to make this recipe contains good amounts of healthy protein.

This particular recipe allows you to make a total of 5 servings and contains 434 calories. Of this recipe 39 grams is protein, 49 grams is carbs and 6 grams is fat.

Ingredients

2 Cups Uncooked Quinoa
24 Ounces Cooked Chicken Breast
2 Cups Salsa
1 Cup Chopped Raw Onion
1 Diced Jalapeno To Taste (Is Optional)

Instructions

Step 1 – In a saucepan place the quinoa with 4 cups of water and bring to the boil. As soon as the water is boiling vigorously turn the heat down to a medium to low level and allow the quinoa to continue cooking in the water until only a small amount of water is left.

Step 2 – Remove the quinoa from the heat and allow to stand covered for 10 minutes. Any water that's remaining will soak into the quinoa.

Step 3 – In a large mixing bowl place the cooked chicken, salsa and onion and stir in the cooked and cooled quinoa. You can also add Jalapenos if you wish. Now divide the mixture evenly into five separate servings and place in containers. Then freeze or place in the refrigerator.

Recipe 3 – Scallop Ceviche

For anyone who loves seafood they're going to love this particular recipe. It is very low in calories, but has a large amount of protein and tastes absolutely amazing.

This recipe will provide you with a total of 3 servings and each serving contains 241 calories. Of this recipe 26 grams is protein, 7 grams is carbs and 10 grams is fat.

Ingredients

1lb Bay Scallops (These scallops are much smaller than other types you can get, normally they are about the size of a marble)
Juice of 6 Limes (You need enough juice to cover the scallops. Also if you want you can use lemon juice instead)
½ Large Red Onion Chopped
1 Medium Tomato
1 Stalk of Celery
2 Tablespoons of Capers
2 Tablespoons of Olive Oil
Pinch of Sea Salt
1 Tablespoon Ground Black Pepper (or enough to taste)

Instructions

Step 1 – Place the scallops into a shallow bowl and pour over the lime juice.

Step 2 – Cover the bowl, place in the refrigerator and leave for between 4 to 8 hours. You could even leave them in the refrigerator over night if you wish.

Step 3 – After the scallops have soaked in the lime juice remove them from the bowl and drain most of the remaining juice.

Step 4 – Now take the onion, tomato and celery and dice into pieces then add these to the scallops along with the capers, salt, olive oil and pepper. Place the bowl (covered) back in the refrigerator and leave for another few hours before serving it cold.

Dinner Recipes

Recipe 1 – Mediterranean Rice

This particular recipe helps to turn a tin of tuna into something a little more extraordinary.

This particular recipe will make only one serving and contains between 590 and 600 calories. Each serving of this recipe contains 30 to 32 grams of protein, 80 grams of carbs and 10 to 16 grams of fat.

Ingredients

1 Can of Tuna
100grams (3/4 Cup) Basmati Rice
¼ or 1/3 Red Onion
Half Lemon Squeezed
¼ or 1/3 Avocado
Salt & Pepper To Taste (Optional)

Instructions

Step 1 – Place the basmati rice into a pan of boiling water and allow to cook for between 15 and 20 minutes.

Step 2 – When cooked, allow the rice to cool before placing into a mixing bowl.

Step 3 – Now take the red onion and cut into strips and add to the rice.

Step 4 – Drain the tuna oil and add to the rice and onions.

Step 5 – Cut up the avocado into small squares and add to rice, onion and tuna and add the squeezed lemon juice.

Step 6 – Mix all the ingredients in the bowl together thoroughly and taste. Add salt and pepper as required.

Recipe 2 – Swedish Beef Patties With Onions

This isn't only a very easy recipe to make but won't cost a great deal. Use this recipe to make several servings you can enjoy through the week.

Each serving of this recipe contains 300 calories and contains 16 grams of protein, 20 grams of carbs and 16.9 grams of fat.

Ingredients

2 Cold Boiled Potatoes
1lb Lean Ground Minced Beef
Salt & White Pepper To Taste
3 Tablespoons of Water
2 Tablespoons of Butter or Margarine
2 Large Onions Sliced

Instructions

Step 1 – Take the cold boiled potatoes and mash them.

Step 2 – Take the mashed potatoes and combine these with the minced beef and then add salt and pepper to taste along with water. Continue to work the mixture until it becomes smooth then shape into patties.

Step 3 – Warm the skillet on a moderate heat and place a tablespoon of butter or margarine and add the onions. Cook the onions until they turn a golden brown.

Step 4 – Now take the onions out of the skillet and place on a hot plate.

Step 5 – Take the remaining tablespoon of butter/margarine and place in the skillet and cook the patties over a moderate heat until they're brown on both sides. Also make sure they are cooked through.

Step 6 – Once the patties are cooked serve on a plate with the onions and vegetables of your choice.

NB: Serve the onions on top of the patties.

Recipe 3 – Lemon Thyme Roast Chicken

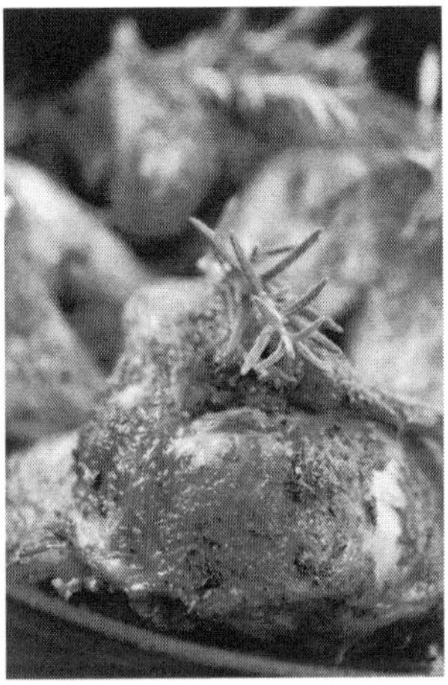

You can serve this meal with just about anything you want from brown rice and salad to whole boiled potatoes and roasted vegetables.

Each serving of this roast chicken contains 165 calories. Also each serving contains 25 grams of protein, 1 gram of carbs and 6 grams of fat.

Ingredients

4lb 8oz Roasting Chicken
1 Teaspoon Freshly Ground Black Pepper
½ Teaspoon Salt
2 Large Lemons
6 Garlic Cloves Peeled
6 x 4" Fresh Thyme Sprigs or 2 Teaspoon Dried Thyme Leaves
Additional Sprigs of Thyme To Act As A Garnish

Instructions

Step 1 – Preheat the oven to a temperature of 350 degrees Fahrenheit (180 degrees Centigrade).

Step 2 – Whilst the oven is heating up sprinkle the chicken cavities with ½ teaspoon of pepper and ¼ teaspoon of salt.

Step 3 – Next on a work surface roll the lemons pressing down on them slightly with the heel of your hand. Continue to press lightly on the lemons until they become soft.

Step 4 – Now take a skewer or a toothpick and pierce each lemon 15 times to a depth of about 1 inch. Now take the pierced lemons, 5 garlic cloves and the thyme and place these inside the chicken. As for the other clove of garlic this should be placed in the smaller cavity to the rear. Then truss the chicken up.

Step 5 – Sprinkle over the chicken the remaining pepper and salt and place it breast side up on to a rack in a large roasting plan. Place in the oven and cook for between 2 and 2 ¼ hours, or until the chicken is cooked through.

The juices should run clear when the chicken is thoroughly cooked. However to ensure it's properly cooked insert a meat thermometer into the thickest part of the chicken thigh. If the temperature registers 180 degrees this tells you the chicken is cooked and can now be removed from the oven.

Step 6 – After removing the chicken from the oven allow it to stand for 10 minutes before carving. First remove the skin and discard before removing the lemons, garlic and thyme. Once you've done you're now able to carve the chicken and serve.

Step 7 – Serve each portion to your guests with a sprig of thyme.

Recipe 4 – Cheesy Baked Eggplant

If you haven't tried cooking eggplant before then you may want to give this recipe a try. As well as being a very healthy vegetarian option you'll find this is a very tasty dish.

Each serving, which is around 1/3 of the pan, contains 358 calories. Plus each serving of this recipe contains 19 grams of protein, 32 grams of carbs and 19 grams of fat.

Ingredients

1 Eggplant
16oz Tin Diced Tomatoes
2 x 8oz Tins Tomato Sauce
6oz Cheese (Cheddar or Swiss is fine)
Medium Onion Chopped
Oregano To Taste
2 Teaspoons Salt
Italian Seasoning To Taste
Basil To Taste
Thyme To Taste
2 to 3 Teaspoons Garlic Powder or Salt
½ Teaspoon Freshly Ground Black Pepper

Instructions

Step 1 – Take the eggplant and peel before then cutting into slices. Then liberally sprinkle salt over all the slices and allow to sit for ½ hour.

Step 2 – Take some paper towel after the ½ hour has passed and use this to mop up any liquid that has formed. Then thoroughly rinse the slices of eggplant in water.

Step 3 – Now take each slice and cut into quarters and place one layer of them in the bottom of a baking tray that measures 9 x 13.

Step 4 – Over the layer of eggplant slices pour ½ tin of diced tomato along with 1 tin of tomato sauce and layer slices of cheese on top. Then season with a little salt and pepper and the oregano, Italian seasoning, basil, thyme, garlic powder/salt and black pepper.

Step 5 – Repeat the same again before then placing into a preheated oven with a temperature of 350 degrees Fahrenheit (180 degrees Centigrade). Then cook for 45 minutes. Once cooked serve.

Snack Recipes

Recipe 1 – Healthy Chocolate Raspberry Dessert

Each serving you make contains 159 calories and each serving is made up of 9 grams of protein, 21 grams of carbs and 5 grams of fat.

Ingredients

2 Cups Raspberries (Fresh or Frozen)
2 Cups Fat Free Plain Yogurt
1.5 Oz Dark Chocolate

Instructions

Step 1 – If you're using frozen raspberries in this recipe then first you need to gently defrost them in the microwave. Allow them to defrost until they reach around room temperature.

Step 2 – Now slowly melt the chocolate. You can either do this by placing the chocolate in a bowl in the microwave or by placing in a bowl on top of a saucepan of boiling water.

Step 3 – Once the chocolate has melted, remove the bowl from the microwave or the hob and allow the mixture to cool slightly. Then gently fold the raspberries and yogurt until all ingredients are well blended.

Step 4 – Now take the mixture and pour into either bowls or cups and place in the refrigerator to chill.

Step 5 – Once the mixture has chilled sufficiently take out of the refrigerator and top with some fresh raspberries or blueberries or some crushed almonds or pistachios and then serve.

NB: If you are looking to add more muscle mass then you need to add a few more calories to this recipe. The best way to add an additional 60 calories to each serving is to replace the plain yogurt with Greek yogurt.

Recipe 2 – Whey Brownie

As well as being very simple to make these brownies are very tasty.

Each of these brownies comprises a total of 104 calories and each one is made up of 22 grams of protein, 1 gram of carbs and 1 gram of fat. Also you can make sure that you are getting your full dietary requirements when eating these by topping with something like peanut butter or have them with some oatmeal in the morning.

This particular recipe enables you to make four brownies.

Ingredients

4 Scoops of Whey Protein Any Flavor You Like
7 oz Water or Coffee (Use Coffee To make A Mocha Brownie)

Instructions

Step 1 – Preheat the oven to a temperature of 400 degrees Fahrenheit (200 degrees Centigrade).

Step 2 – In a mixing bowl place 4 scoops of whey protein and add the water or coffee.

Step 3 – Whisk the ingredients together until a smooth mixture is created. Then scoop the mixture on to a baking tray or into a silicone cup cake tray that you've first coated with non-stick cooking spray.

Step 4 – Place the mixture into the oven and cook for 15 minutes or until you notice the mixture has become harder. Once cooked through remove from oven and let the brownies cool before removing from the tray.

Recipe 3 – Blueberry Muffins

What could be healthier than these as a snack you can enjoy at any time of the day as part of your strength training diet and nutrition regime?

The number of calories that each muffin contains is 476. Each of these muffins contains 39 grams of protein, 53 grams of carbs and 12 grams of fat.

Ingredients

¾ Cup Oats
1 Cup Egg Whites
½ Cup Blueberries (Fresh or Frozen is Acceptable)
60 gram Peanut Butter (To Be Added After The Muffins Are Baked)

Instructions

Step 1 - Pre heat the oven to a temperature of 350 degrees Fahrenheit (180 degrees Centigrade).

Step 2 – Whilst the oven is heating up in a bowl place the oats, egg whites and blueberries and mix thoroughly together.

Step 3 – Now pour the mixture into a muffin tin, which has been sprayed with some non-stick cooking oil first, and place the muffin tray in the oven and leave the muffins to cook for 30 minutes.

Step 4 – When 30 minutes has passed, remove the muffins from the oven before allowing them to cool and top them with peanut butter if you want.

Recipe 4 – Peanut Butter Cookies

These can be enjoyed at any time and provide you with a sweet tasting but healthy snack between meals.

Jason Scotts

This recipe enables you to make a total of 36 cookies and each one of these cookies contains 96.73 calories. Plus each cookie contains 4.17 grams of protein, 10.09 grams of carbs and 4.99 grams of fat.

Ingredients

2 ½ Cups of Oat Flour
2. 69.8 grams Protein Powder
½ Teaspoon Salt
½ Teaspoon Baking Powder
½ Teaspoon Apple Sauce
1 ½ Cups Peanut Butter
½ Cup Honey
2 Egg Whites

Instructions

Step 1 – Turn the oven on and set at a temperature of 375 degrees Fahrenheit (190 degrees Centigrade).

Step 2 – Into a bowl place the flour, protein powder, salt and baking soda and place to one side.

Step 3 – In another bowl place the apple sauce and peanut butter and mix together, then add the honey and mix well before then adding to this mixture the egg whites and beat all these ingredients together well.

Step 4 – Now take the dry ingredients and mix these into the peanut butter mixture until a smooth dough is created.

Step 5 – On to a greased baking sheet drop teaspoons of the dough and flatten each.

Step 6 – Now place the baking sheet into the oven and cook for between 10 and 15 minutes or until the dough has turned a light brown color. Then remove from oven and allow to cool.

Chapter 7 – Strength Training Diet & Nutrition Tips

Here's some strength training diet and nutrition tips you may find helpful and will ensure you keep on track with yours.

Tip 1 – Avoid eating any foods that are highly processed. So avoid eating anything that comes in a bag or box. Although the label may recommend they are suitable, these products tend to contain high levels of sugar and saturated fats.

Tip 2 – Whenever you can, buy fresh food that 's grown locally at a farmers market for example. Not only are you ensuring the food you're buying is the freshest but will tend not to have been treated with a wide array of chemicals.

Tip 3 – As a follow on from tip 2 try to focus on using foods in your diet that are free of pesticides and free from antibiotic or hormone animal protein. So eat as much organic food as you possibly can.

Tip 4 – If you can, choose fish that 's been caught wild rather than raised on a farm.

Tip 5 – Whenever possible try to avoid drinking or eating anything out of plastic.

Tip 6 – It's important to increase your fiber intake, as this will help you to eliminate waste containing toxins and other chemicals from your body more effectively. Plus fiber will help you to maintain a regular toilet schedule.

Tip 7 – When it comes to shopping for food you should be aiming to do yours at least twice a week to ensure everything you eat is as fresh as possible. The fresher the food the more nutrients, minerals and vitamins they'll contain.

Tip 8 – You should continue to chew anything you eat until it has turned to puree before swallowing. Doing this will not only help your body to absorb much more quickly but also will help you to feel fuller for longer.

Tip 9 – Whenever possible eat raw food. However avoid eating chicken, turkey, pork or lamb raw as these contain a bacterium that can cause quite dangerous food poisoning.

Tip 10 - Make sure you include plenty of green vegetables into your diet.

Tip 11 – Although grains are important to a diet you shouldn't eat too many of these and if at all possible cut them out from your diet completely.

Tip 12 – When it comes to wanting to get plenty of carbs, the best foods to eat for this are potatoes, buckwheat and quinoa.

Tip 13 – You should try to drink at least half your bodyweight in ounces of water each day. Therefore if you way 128 lbs you should be drinking at least 64 ounces of water each day.

Tip 14 – If you can, make sure you include digestive enzymes and probiotics into your diet. Food that is best to get probiotics from, other than the yogurts, are Kimchi and live Sauerkraut.

Tip 15 – For those of you who are trying to lose weight as well as increase strength try to cut down on how much fruit you eat.

Tip 16 – Make sure during the winter months you take a supplement of between 5 and 6 grams of Vitamin C each day. Not only will Vitamin C help to boost your immune system but also help to prevent you suffering from fatigue.

Tip 17 – We all like sugar but it's important to try and completely eliminate it from your diet. It may taste nice but it doesn't help your body to work more effectively.

Tip 18 – Avoid overcooking your food, this will prevent it from losing the vital nutrients, minerals and vitamins your body needs.

Tip 19 – Make sure you include foods into your strength training diet and nutrition program that contain good amounts of Omega 3 Fatty Acids in them.

Tip 20 – Having a cup or two of black coffee each day won't actually do you any harm. In fact drinking it can help to increase how much fat your body burns off as long as you drink it at the right times.

Tip 21 – For those who like to train first thing in the morning before they eat and want to gain muscle then I would recommend taking 10 grams of BCAA around 15 to 30 minutes before the workout commences.

Tip 22 – Make sure you drink freshly squeezed vegetable juice each day. Not only do these provide you with a great source of nutrients but also live enzymes.

Tip 23 – If you're having problems with your digestive system then add some apple cider vinegar into some of your meals, as it will help to improve it.

Tip 24 – As well as rotating what you eat each day, don't be afraid to try out some new foods whenever possible. For example instead of cooking some meals with chicken choose to use quail instead.

Tip 25 – The oils I would recommend you use for cooking food with is either red palm, coconut or macadamia oil.

Tip 26 – When it comes to cooking eggs make sure you change the way in which you cook them regularly. So one day you should have them poached or hard boiled, then another day go for scrambled or eggs over easy. By doing this you are helping to reduce the risk of you suffering from any possible food allergies.

Other Killer Resources

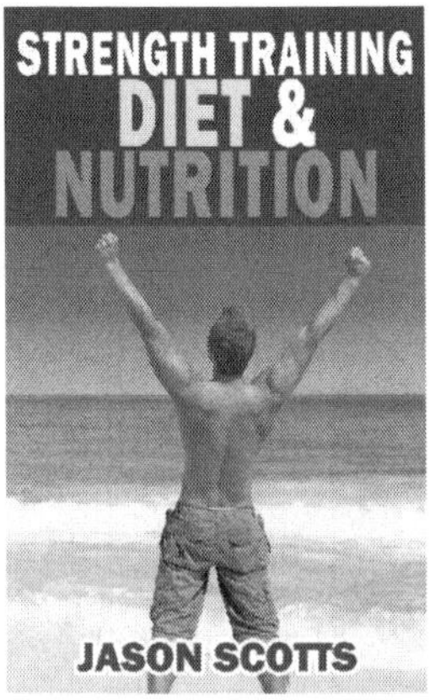

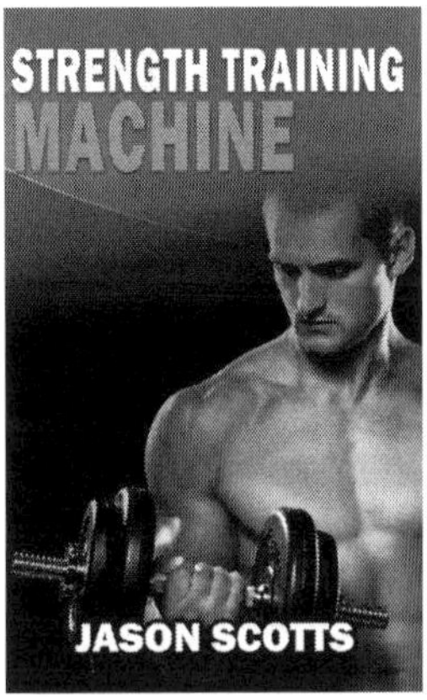

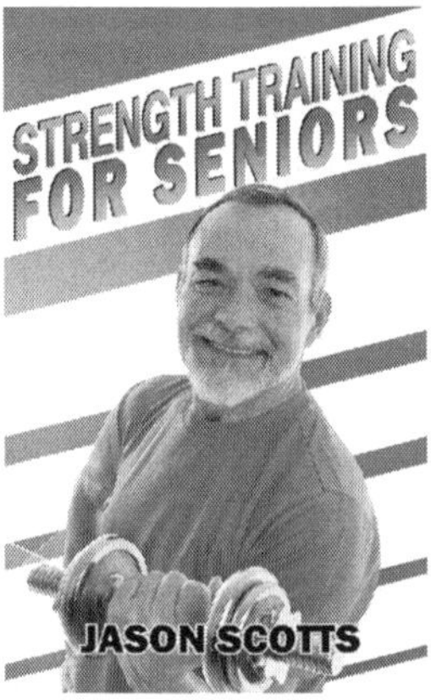

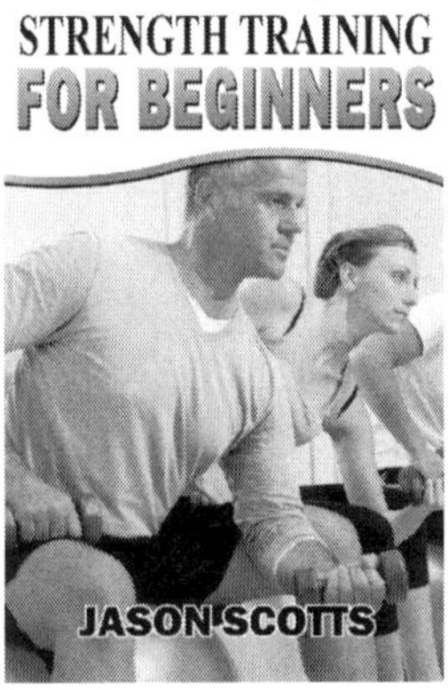

15620234R00028

Printed in Great Britain
by Amazon